LOW POTASSIUM COOKBOOK

Healthy Low Potassium Recipes to Aid Combat with Hyperkalemia

Table of Contents

Introduction *4*

Ginger Mustard Lamb 6

Beef 'N' Rice 8

Herbaceous Omelette 10

Peppery Beef Steak 13

Herbs Beef Burger 16

Beef Meatballs 18

Beef Steak Sandwich 22

Beef Tacos 24

Simple 'N' Basic Turkey Meatloaf 27

Fish Croquettes 29

Baked Trout Fillets 31

Shrimps Eggs Salad 34

Shrimps Crabs Supreme 37

Baked Lemon Crab Cakes 39

Baked Flaky Fish Fillets 42

Rotini Tuna Salad 44

Beef Vegetables Soup 47

Egg Noodles Chicken Soup 49

Fruity Omelette 52

Meat Stuffed Green Peppers 55

Jalapeno Pepper Chicken 58

Crispy Lemon Chicken 61

Old Style Rice and Chicken 64

Chicken and Celery Salad 67

Simple Vegetables and Chicken Salad 70

Spring Onions and Herbs Chicken Curry 72

Chicken and Vegetables Stew.. 75

Stir Fry Vegetables Chicken 78

Simple 'N' Basic Pork Chops 80

Pan Pork Sausage... 82

Conclusion *84*

Introduction

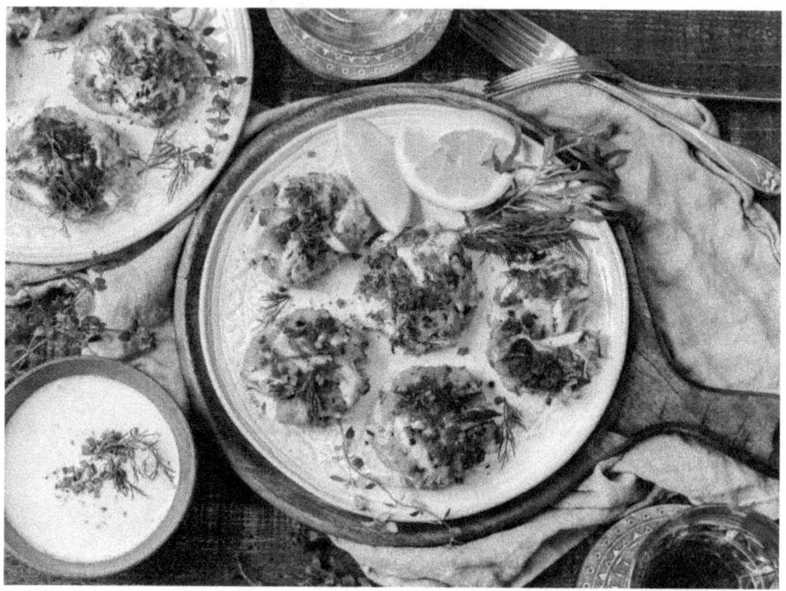

Have you been diagnosed with high potassium levels in your blood (Hyperkalemia)? Here are 30 nutritious Low Potassium Homemade Recipes for you.

This book is specifically designed for persons who have been told by their doctors that they have Hyperkalemia or similar medical conditions which warrants them to limit their potassium in.

Now, let us take a closer look at what this book has to offer:

- Low Potassium Recipe Cookbook has 30 nutritious and delicious low potassium homemade recipes specifically designed for persons with high levels of potassium levels in the blood or similar conditions medically. These recipes are done from basic ingredients that are used in your kitchen or backyard cooking daily or they can be easily found in the grocery store. These recipes include Side dishes, Main dishes, Desserts and Beverages.

- Eating right and consuming the right nutrition will help in the reduction of further damage to your health and eventually healing you. The right diet will help to minimize the symptoms, also prevent weight loss and malnutrition. People with Hyperkalemia (high potassium levels in the blood) probably need to limit nutrients such as phosphorus and sodium too in their diet. Saturated and Trans-fat should be limited too. Low Potassium Recipe Cookbook will help you to achieve these goals.

Ginger Mustard Lamb

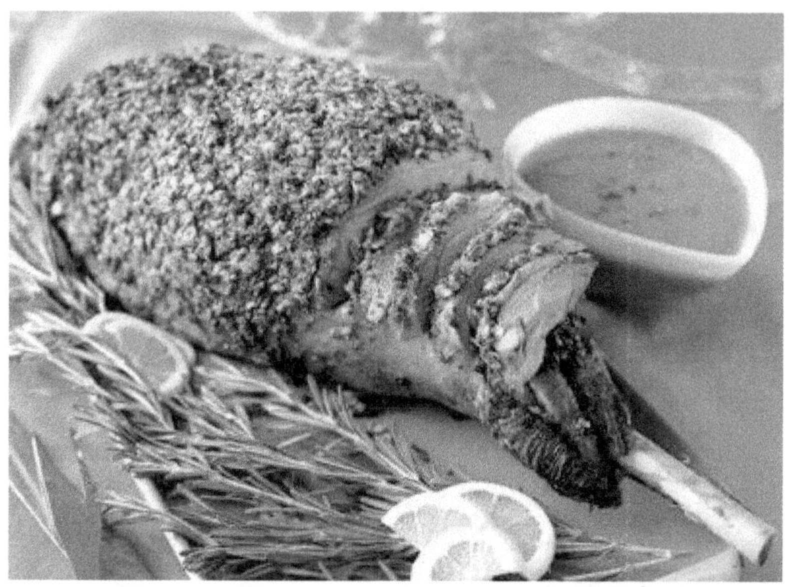

This delicious lamb dish is succulent, flavorful and best of all easy to make.

Serves: 4

Time: 8 hrs. 30 mins.

Ingredients

- ¼ cup vegetable oil
- 1 ½ tbsp. garlic powder
- 3 tsp. dry mustard

- 1 leg of lamb (trimmed for roasting)

Directions

1. Combine oil, mustard and ginger powder together well.

2. Now, put and coat the lamb legs well with the mixture. Once the lamb legs are coated well with mixture, refrigerate the lamb legs for at least 6 to 8 hours or overnight.

3. Remove the lamb from refrigerate and place on barbeque spit.

4. Keep basting the meat continuously with the marinade and roast the lamb legs for around 30 (internal temperature should be 170 degrees F). Enjoy!

Nutritional Content:

Calories: 289

Potassium: 423 mg

Fat: 6g

Protein: 24g

Beef 'N' Rice

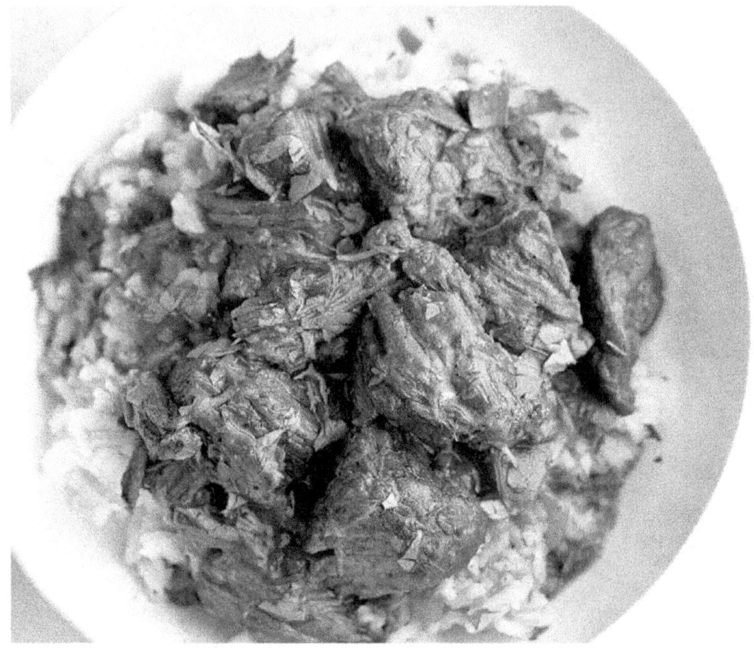

Enjoy this delicious beef and rice dish in under an hour.

Serves: 4

Time: 30 mins.

Ingredients

- vegetable oil, 2 tbsp.
- ground beef, lean, 1 pound
- onion, 1 cup, chopped

- rice, 2 cups, cooked
- chili con carne seasoning powder, 1 ½ tsp.
- black pepper, ⅛ tsp.
- sage, ½ tsp.

Directions

1. Start by heating the oil.

2. Next step is to add the beef and onions. Cook the beef, while stirring, until browns.

3. Once the beef browns, add the rice, sage and chili con carne seasoning powder. Mix everything together well.

4. Remove from the heat, close the lid then let stand for at least 10 to 15 minutes.

Nutritional Content:

Calories: 360

Potassium: 27mg

Fat: 14g

Protein: 23g

Herbaceous Omelette

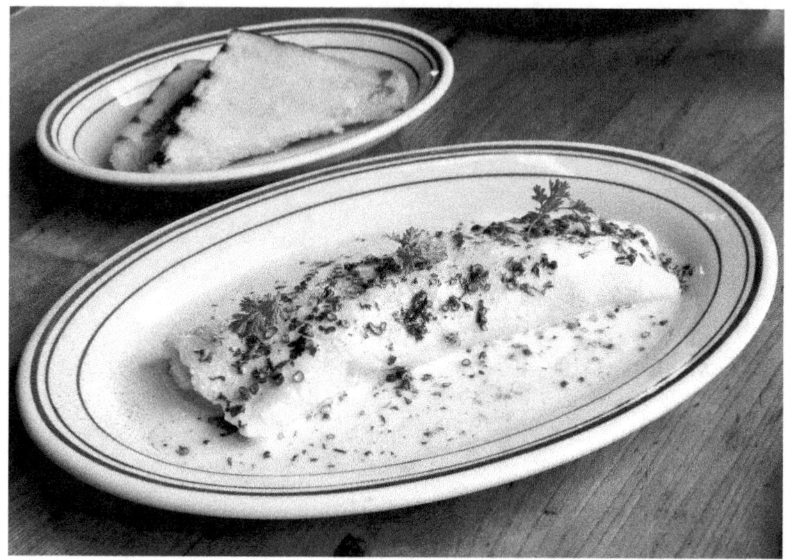

This delicious omelette can be whipped up in minutes to create the perfect busy morning meal.

Serves: 2

Time: 15 mins.

Ingredients

- vegetable oil, 1½ tsp.
- onion, 1 tbsp., chopped
- eggs, 4
- water, 2 tbsp.

- basil, ¼ tsp.

- tarragon, ⅛ tsp.

- parsley, ¼ tsp. (optional)

Directions

1. Take a bowl and beat the eggs. Now, add spices and water.

2. Now, heat the oil in an 8" frying pan over medium heat. Once the oil is hot, add and sauté the spring onions. Remove from the pan.

3. Now, add your mixture to a hot frying pan on medium heat.

4. As the omelette sets, lift with the help of a spatula to allow the omelette to cook on all parts.

5. When the omelette is completely set, add the sautéed spring onions to the top of the omelette and remove from pan to a serving dish.

Nutritional Content:

Calories: 195

Potassium: 157mg

Fat: 15g

Protein: 14g

Peppery Beef Steak

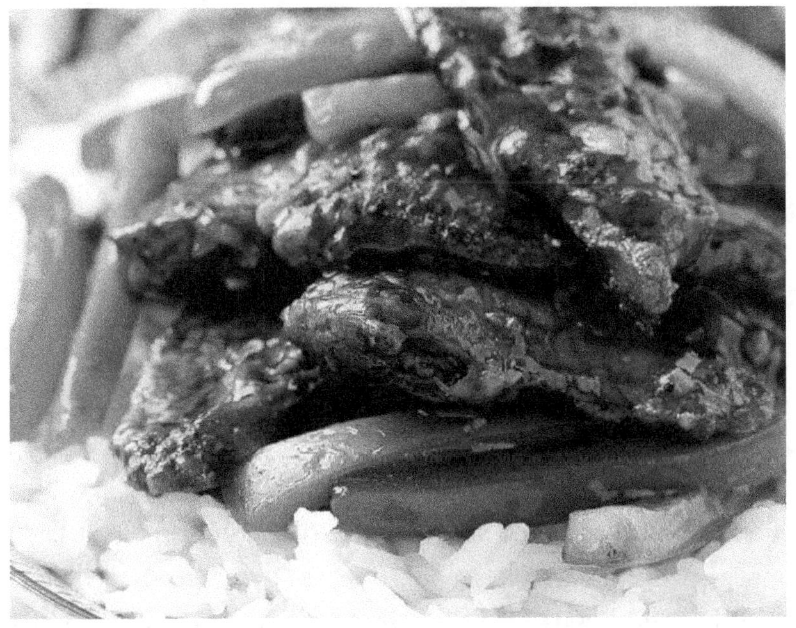

Enjoy a spicy bite with this Peppery Beef Steak.

Serves: 4

Time: 30 mins.

Ingredients

- chopped steak, 1 pound
- onion, 1 small, chopped
- green pepper, ½ cup, chopped
- black pepper

- egg, 1
- vegetable oil, 1 tbsp.
- water, ½ cup
- corn starch, 1 tbsp.

Directions

1. First step is to take a bowl and mix egg, onions, pepper, green pepper and meat together well. Once mixed well, form the mixture into patties.

2. Next step is to take a skillet and heat the oil. Once hot, place the patties in the skillet and cook on both the sides.

3. Now, add a half of your water then simmer for about 15 minutes before remove the patties.

4. Now add the remaining water and corn starch. Let it simmer while constantly stirring to thicken the gravy.

5. Final step is to pour the gravy over the steak and serve hot.

Nutritional Content:

Calories: 249

Potassium: 366 mg

Fat: 57g

Protein: 22g

Herbs Beef Burger

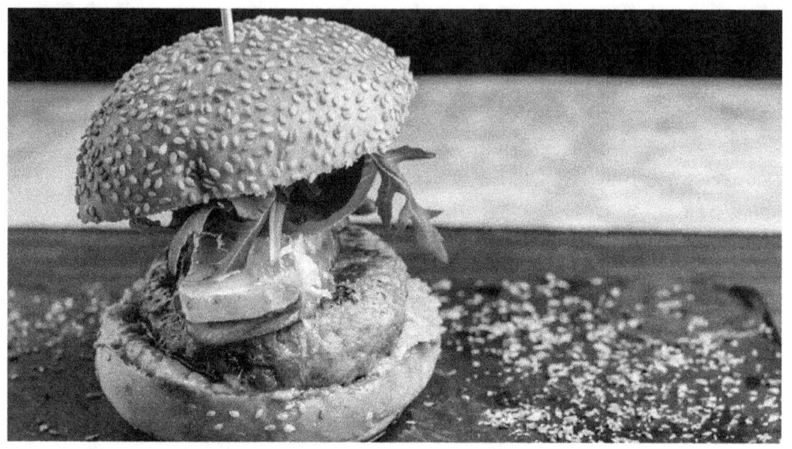

This delicious burger will blow your mind with its savory flavor.

Serves: 4

Time: 30 mins

Ingredients

- 1 pound lean ground beef
- 1 tbsp. lemon juice
- 1 tbsp. parsley flakes
- ¼ tsp. black pepper
- ¼ tsp. ground thyme
- ¼ tsp. oregano

Directions

1. Start by mixing all the **Ingredients** thoroughly in a medium or large bowl.

2. Next step is to shape the mixture into patties. Please make the patties about ¾ inches thick.

3. Now, take a skillet or broiler pan and grease it with a little oil.

4. Final step is to broil the patties about 3 inches from the heat for about 10 to 15 minutes, turning once.

Nutritional Content:

Calories: 171

Potassium: 289mg

Fat: 10g

Protein: 20g

Beef Meatballs

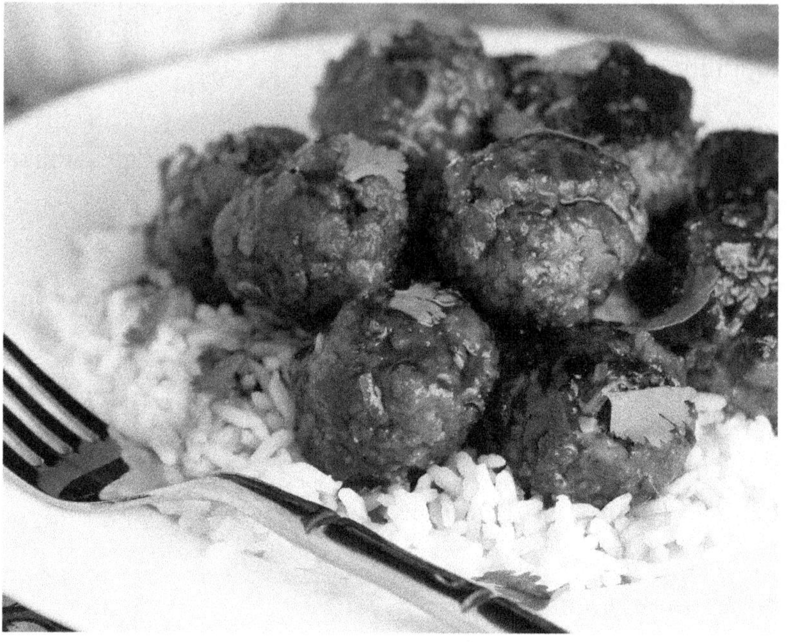

These meatballs are juicy and filled with flavor.

Serves: 18

Time: 40 mins.

Ingredients

Meatballs:

- 1 pound lean ground turkey
- onions, ¼ cup, finely chopped

- lemon juice, 1 tbsp.

- poultry seasoning, 1 tsp. (without salt)

- black pepper, 1 tsp.

- dry mustard, ¼ tsp.

- onion powder, ¾ tsp.

- Italian seasoning, 1 tsp.

- granulated sugar, 1 tsp.

- Tabasco® sauce, 1 tsp.

Sauce:

- vegetable oil, ¼ cup

- all-purpose flour, 2 tbsp.

- onion powder, 1 tsp.

- vinegar, 2 tsp.

- sugar, 2 tsp.

- Tabasco® sauce, 1 tsp.

- Water, 2-3 cups

Directions

Meatballs:

1. Preheat the oven to 425°F.

2. Next step is to take a bowl and mix all
the **Ingredients** together well.

3. Once the mixture is ready, shape the meatballs. Each meatball should have one tbsp. of meat mixture.

4. Now, place the meatballs in a baking dish and bake them for about 20 minutes or until well done.

5. Final step is to remove the meatballs from the oven and combine them with the sauce. Keep the meatballs warm until you are ready to serve.

Sauce:

6. Start by taking a saucepan, placing on heat and combining oil and flour in it. Keep stirring.

7. Now, add vinegar, sugar, onion powder, mild sauce and water

8. Once you add all the **Ingredients**, return the pan to heat and continue stirring until the sauce thickens.

Nutritional Content:

Calories: 76

Potassium: 70mg

Fat: 6g

Protein: 5g

Beef Steak Sandwich

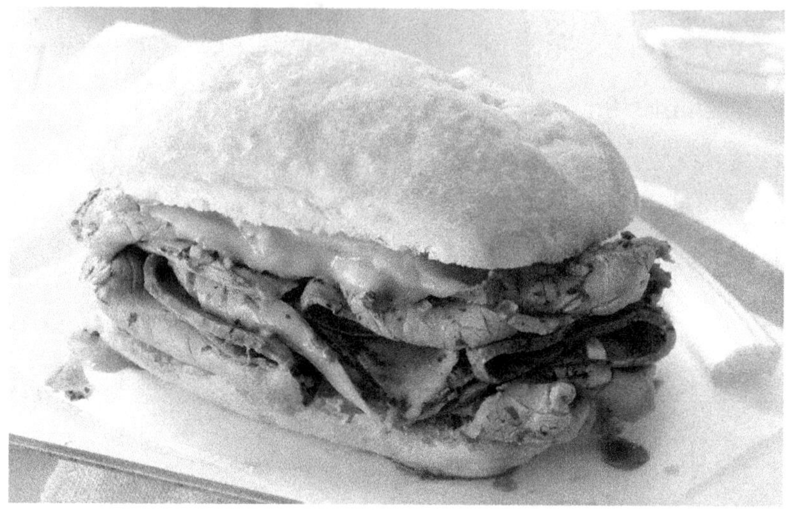

This sandwich is perfect for picnics and brown bag lunches.

Serves: 4

Time: 35 mins.

Ingredients

- 4 chopped steaks (4-ounces each)
- 1 tbsp. lemon juice
- 1 tbsp. Italian seasoning
- 1 tbsp. black pepper
- 1 tbsp. vegetable oil
- 1 medium onion, sliced into rings

- 4 hoagie rolls, sliced

Directions

1. Start by taking a bowl and combining the meat, Italian seasoning, black pepper and lemon juice in it.

2. Next step is to take a frying pan and heat the oil over medium heat.

3. Next step is to brown the beef steaks on both the sides until they are tender. Drain on the paper towels.

4. Now, reduce the heat and in the same pan, add onions and sauté them until they are tender.

5. In order to serve, serve open faced on roasted or grilled bread slices.

Nutritional Content:

Calories: 345

Potassium: 200mg

Fat: 21g

Protein: 14g

Beef Tacos

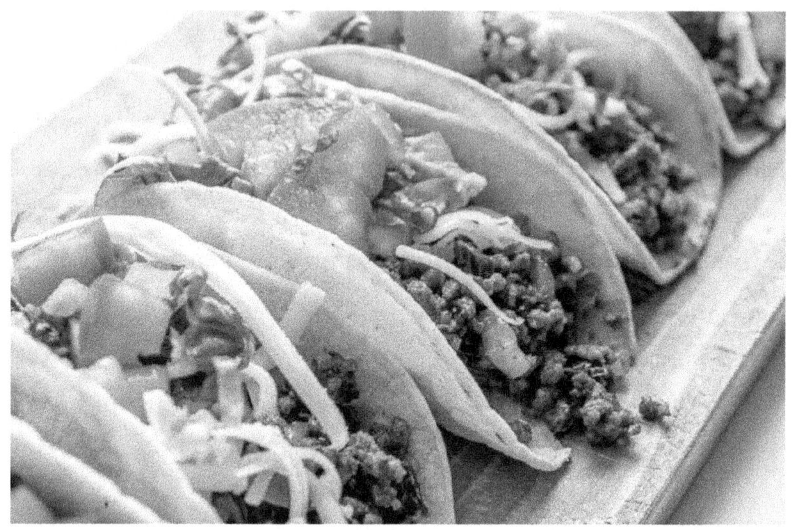

Tasty, hassle – free and delicious. Enjoy these tacos on your next Taco Tuesday.

Serves: 8

Time: 20 mins.

Ingredients

- 2 tbsp. vegetable oil
- 1 ¼ pounds lean ground beef or turkey
- ½ tsp. ground red pepper
- ½ tsp. black pepper

- 1 tsp. Italian seasoning

- 1 tsp. garlic powder

- onion powder, 1 tsp.

- Tabasco® sauce, ½ tsp.

- Nutmeg, ½ tsp.

- taco shells, 1 medium

- lettuce, ½ head, shredded

Directions

1. Start by taking a skillet and heating oil.

2. Next step is to place the meat and all
other **Ingredients** except the tack shells and lettuce in the
skillet.

3. Next, cook the beef until done and all **Ingredients** are
well blended.

4. Final step is to stuff the taco shells with 2 ounces of meat
and top it with the shredded lettuce.

Nutritional Content:

Calories: 176

Potassium: 258mg

Fat: 9g

Protein: 14g

Simple 'N' Basic Turkey Meatloaf

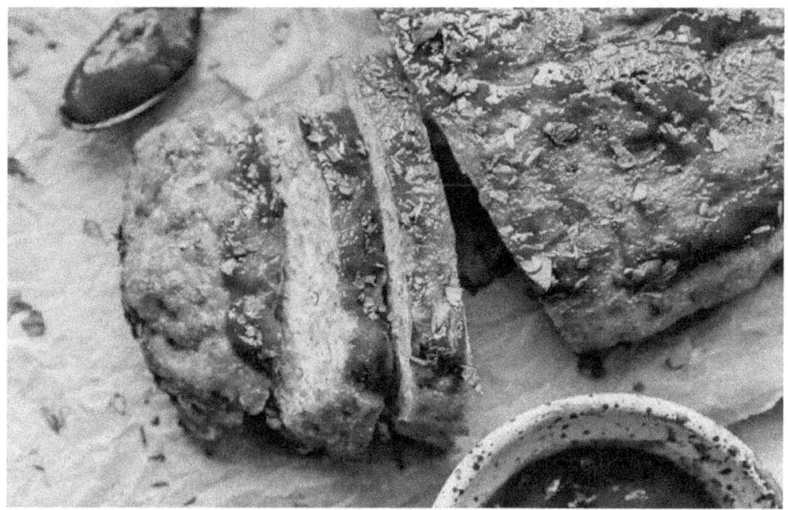

This meatloaf is the perfect evening meal and can be made within an hour.

Serves: 8

Time: 1 hr.

Ingredients

- ground turkey, 1 lb., lean
- egg, 1, white
- lemon juice, 1 tbsp.
- plain breadcrumbs, ½ cup
- onion powder, ½ tsp.

- Italian seasoning, ½ tsp.

- black pepper, ¼ tsp.

- onions, ½ cup, chopped

- green bell pepper, ½ cup, diced

- water, ¼ cup

Directions

1. Start by preheating the oven to 400°F.

2. Add your lemon juice and meat in a bowl.

3. Add all other remaining **Ingredients** to meat and mix well.

4. Finally, place the loaf in a pan and bake for about 45 minutes.

Nutritional Content:

Calories: 110

Potassium: 138mg

Fat: 5g

Protein: 12g

Fish Croquettes

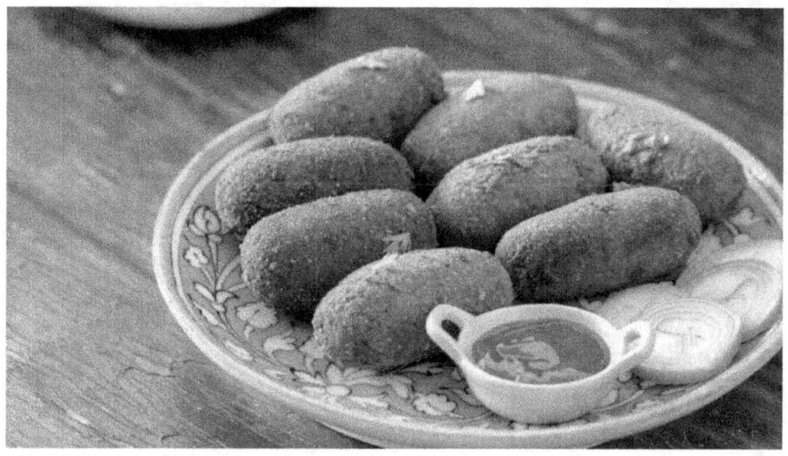

These delicious fish croquettes are perfect for quick lunch or snack.

Serves: 1

Time: 20 mins.

Ingredients

- Salmon, 1 can, water packed
- Eggs, 2, whites
- Onion, ¼ cup, chopped
- black pepper, ½ tsp.
- plain bread crumb, ½ cup
- vegetable oil, 1 tbsp.

- lemon juice, 2 tbsp. (optional)

Directions

1. Start by draining the water from the canned meat.

2. Next step is to take a medium bowl and combine all the **Ingredients** except oil and mix well.

3. Once the mixture is mixed well, Shape the mixture into 8 separate balls, then flatten them into patties.

4. Next step is to take a skillet and heat vegetable oil in it.

5. Once the oil is hot, place the patties in it.

6. Brown the patties on each side. Once the patties are cooked, drain them on paper towels.

Nutritional Content:

Calories: 189

Potassium: 184mg

Fat: 8g

Protein: 14g

Baked Trout Fillets

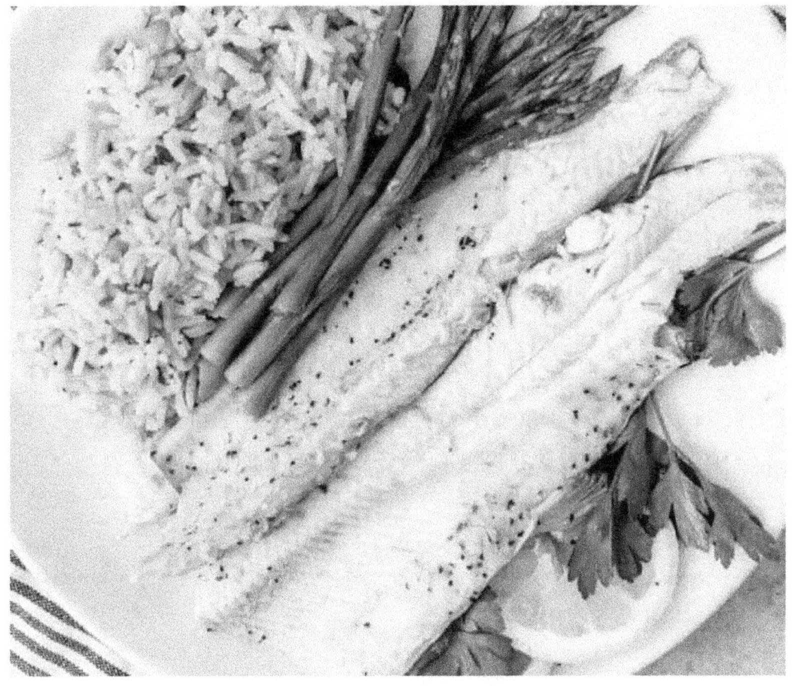

These tasty trout fillets are simple yet juicy.

Serves: 4

Time: 45 mins.

Ingredients

- 4 3-ounce trout filets or any other baking fish
- 1 ½ tsp. black pepper

- 1 tbsp. garlic powder

- 1 ½ tsp. paprika

- ¼ medium green pepper

- 1 small onion

- 1 small lemon

Directions

1. Start by preheating the oven to 375°F.

2. Next step is to place the fish in a greased baking pan or on aluminum foil.

3. Now sprinkle the garlic powder, black pepper, and paprika on both sides of the fish.

4. Also place the chopped spring onions on fish.

5. Now, squeeze the juice of one lemon onto fish.

6. It's now time to bake the fish for 30 minutes.

7. Sprinkle with parmesan cheese after the fish has cooked.

8. Serve hot.

Nutritional Content:

Calories: 164

Potassium: 452mg

Fat: 6g

Protein: 20g

Shrimps Eggs Salad

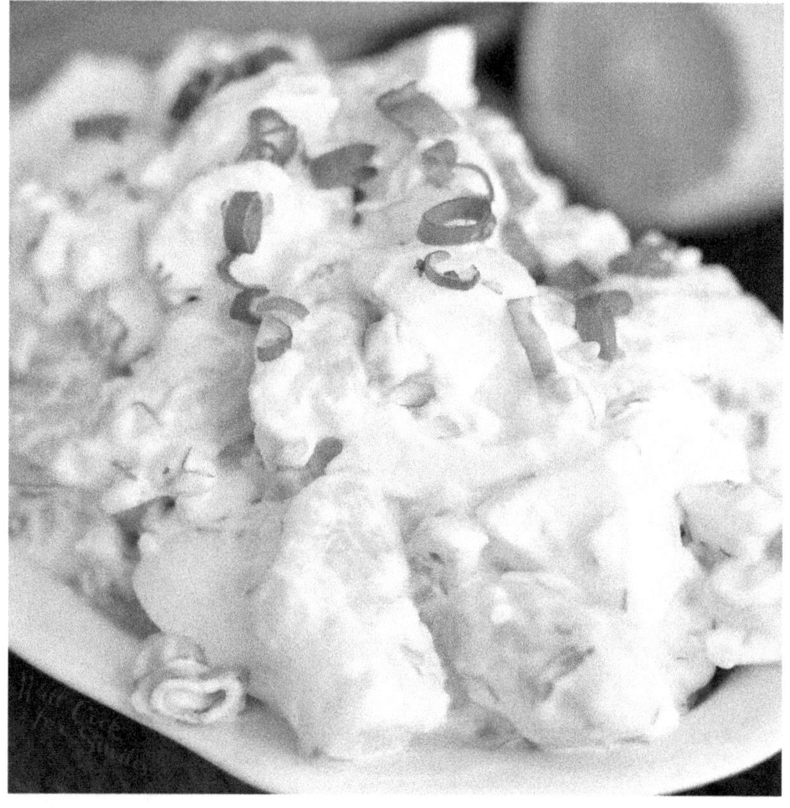

This simple salad is rich, flavorful and delicious.

Serves: 4

Time: 40 mins.

Ingredients

- 1 pound shrimp, boiled, deveined and chopped
- 1 hard-boiled egg, chopped
- 1 tbsp. celery, chopped
- 1 tbsp. green pepper, chopped
- 1 tbsp. onion, chopped
- 2 tbsp. mayonnaise
- 1 tsp. lemon juice
- ½ tsp. chili powder
- ⅛ tsp. Tabasco® or hot sauce
- ½ tsp. dry mustard
- lettuce, chopped or shredded (optional)

Directions

1. Start by combining all the **Ingredients** except lettuce, in a mixing bowl. Mix well.

2. Chill the mixture in the refrigerator for about 30 minutes.

3. To Serve: serve over a lettuce bed.

Nutritional Content:

Calories: 157

Potassium: 233mg

Fat: 5g

Protein: 26g

Shrimps Crabs Supreme

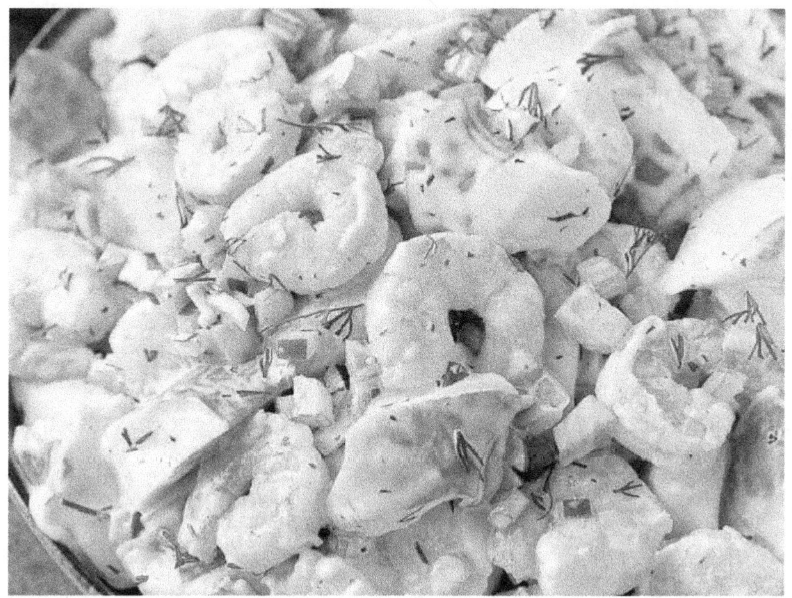

This delicious supreme makes for a simple yet tasty dinner.

Serves: 6

Time: 40 mins.

Ingredients

- 1 c. crabmeat, cooked (boiled)
- 1 c. shrimp, cooked (boiled)
- 4 tbsp. green pepper, chopped
- 2 tbsp. green onions, chopped

- 1 c. celery, chopped

- ½ c. frozen green peas

- ½ tsp. black pepper

- ½ c. mayonnaise

- 1 c. breadcrumbs

Directions

1. Start by preheating the oven to 375ºF.

2. Combine all the **Ingredients** except the breadcrumbs in a bowl.

3. Now, place the mix in a greased casserole dish and top with breadcrumbs.

4. Finally, bake it for about 30 minutes.

Nutritional Content:

Calories: 220

Potassium: 255mg

Fat: 8g

Protein: 16g

Baked Lemon Crab Cakes

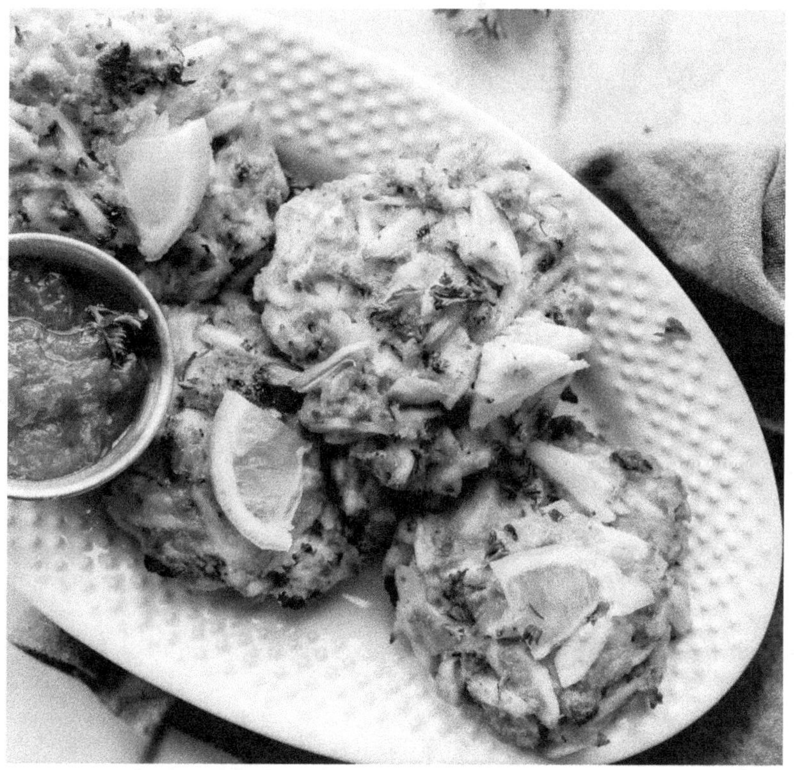

These Lemon Crab Cakes are super tasty and perfect for events.

Serves: 6

Time: 30 mins.

Ingredients

- 1 egg (egg substitute or egg white optional)
- 1/3 c. green or red pepper, finely chopped
- 1/3 c. low sodium crackers
- ¼ c. reduced fat mayonnaise
- 1 tbsp. dry mustard
- 1 tsp. crushed red pepper or black pepper
- 2 tbsp. lemon juice
- 1 tsp. garlic powder
- 2 tbsp. vegetable oil

Directions

1. Start by combining all **Ingredients**.

2. Now, divide the mixture into 6 balls and form patties.

3. Take a pan and heat vegetable oil at medium heat or oven at 350°F.

4. Fry the patties for about 4-5 minutes or bake in the oven for 15 minutes.

5. Serve warm.

Nutritional Content:

Calories: 101

Potassium: 72mg

Fat: 9g

Protein: 2g

Baked Flaky Fish Fillets

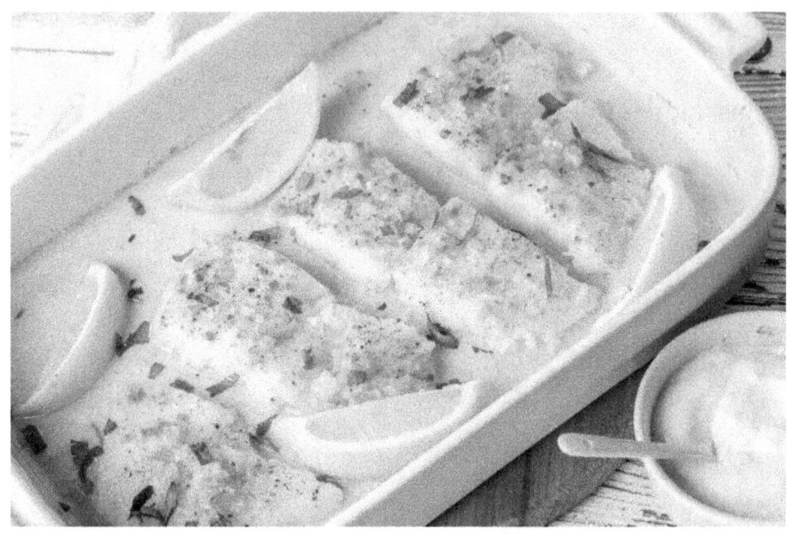

These baked fillets will leave you licking your thumbs.

Serves: 4

Time: 20 mins.

Ingredients

- fish filets, 12-16
- crackers, 20, saltine, unsalted tops, crushed finely
- butter, ¼ cup, unsalted
- dill weed, 2 tsp.
- garlic powder, 1 tsp.

- lemon juice, ¼ cup

Directions

1. Start by preheating the oven to 400ºF.

2. Now, combine the dill, crackers and garlic powder.

3. Next, melt the butter or margarine.

4. Now, roll the fish in the melted butter, then in crumbs and again in the butter mix.

5. Finally, place in the baking pan and bake for about 8 to 10 minutes until the fish is flaky.

Nutritional Content:

Calories: 164

Potassium: 335mg

Fat: 6g

Protein: 21g

Rotini Tuna Salad

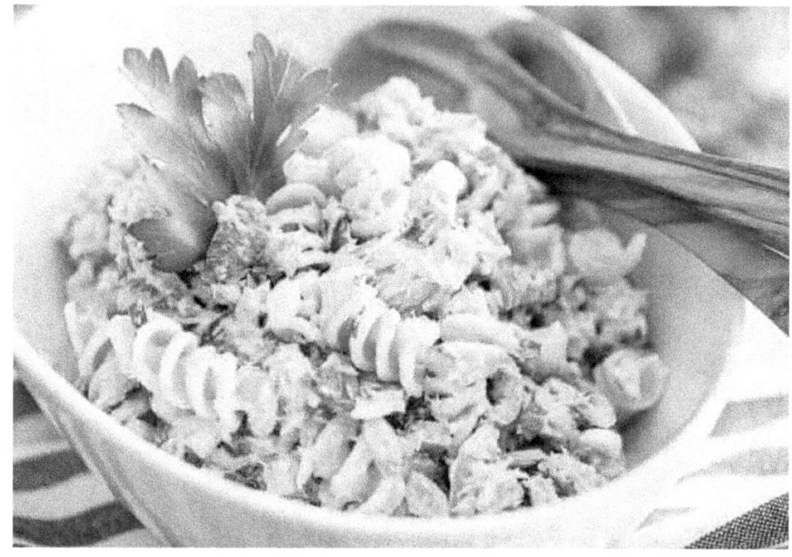

Enjoy this Rotini Tuna Salad for an easy week night dinner.

Serves: 4

Time: 20 mins.

Ingredients

- onion, 2 tbsp., minced
- vegetable cooking spray
- water, 2/3 cup
- curry powder, ¼ tsp.
- black pepper, ¼ tsp.

- chopped fresh parsley (optional)
- 1 9 ¼-ounce with water, low sodium albacore tuna, drained
- cream of mushroom soup, 10 ¾-ounce, canned, undiluted
- rotini, 2 cups, cooked, hot
- green peas, ½ cup frozen thawed

Directions

1. Take a large non-stick skillet and coat it with a spray for cooking. Place the skillet over medium heat.

2. Now, add onions and sauté them until they are tender.

3. Now, take a bowl and combine water, pepper, curry powder and soup. Stir well and then add to skillet.

4. Now, add cooked tuna, rotini and peas. Stir well.

5. Let it cook uncovered over low heat for about 10 minutes, stirring occasionally.

6. Sprinkle with parsley, if desired.

Nutritional Content:

Calories: 269

Potassium: 515mg

Fat: 4g

Protein: 18g

Beef Vegetables Soup

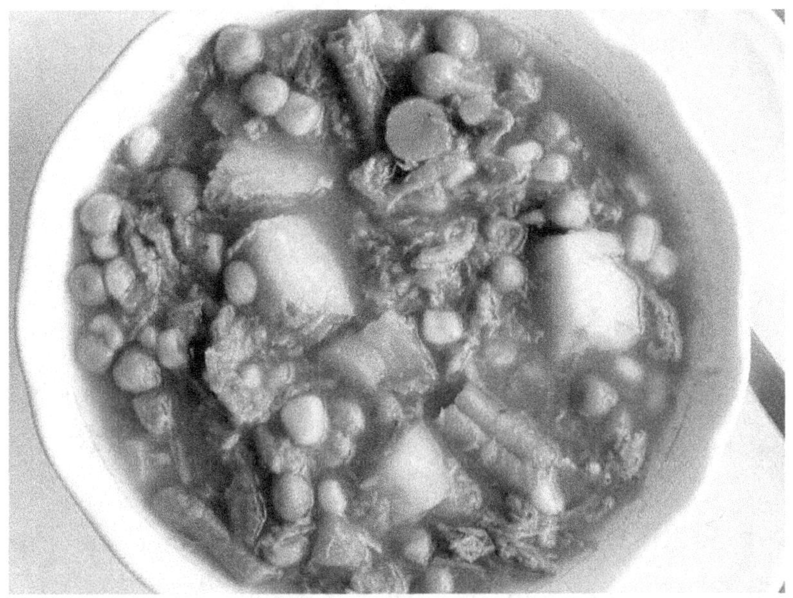

This soup is hassle free, simple and filling.

Serves: 8

Time: 1 hr.

Ingredients

- beef stew, 1 lb.
- Water, 3 ½ c.
- Onions, 1 c., raw, sliced
- green peas, ½ c., frozen

- black pepper, 1 tsp.
- okra, ½ cup, frozen
- basil, ½ tsp.
- carrots, ½ c., frozen, diced
- thyme, ½ tsp.
- corn, ½ c., frozen

Directions

1. Take a large pot and place beef stew, black pepper, onions, basil, thyme and water. Let cook for about 45 minutes.

2. Now, add in your frozen vegetables. Simmer until the meat is tender. If additional water is needed in the soup, you may add ½ cup at a time.

3. Serve hot.

Nutritional Content:

Calories: 190

Potassium: 291mg

Fat: 13g

Protein: 11g

Egg Noodles Chicken Soup

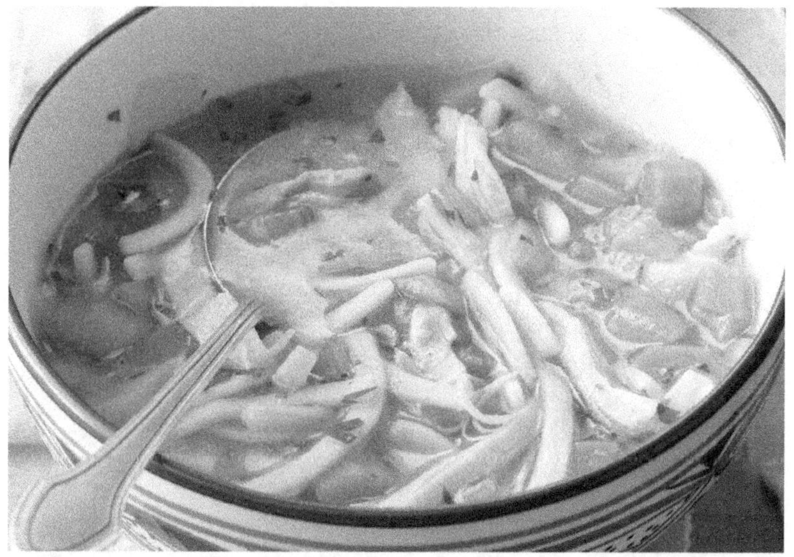

For a tasty and filling soup you can enjoy when you are under the weather try this Egg Noodle and Chicken Soup.

Serves: 8

Time: 1 hr.

Ingredients

- chicken parts, 1lb.
- red pepper, 1 tsp.
- lemon juice, ¼ c.
- caraway seed, 1 tsp.

- Water, 3 ½ c.

- Oregano, 1 tsp.

- poultry seasoning, 1 tsp.

- Sugar, 1 tsp.

- garlic powder, 1 tsp.

- Celery, ½ cup

- onion powder, 1 tsp.

- green pepper, ½ cup

- vegetable oil, 2 tbsp.

- egg noodles, 1 cup

- black pepper, 1 tsp.

Directions

1. Start by rubbing the chicken parts with lemon juice.

2. Take a large pot and combine the chicken, water, garlic powder, poultry seasoning, black pepper, onion powder, vegetable oil, caraway seed, oregano, red pepper and sugar together.

3. Let cook for about 30 minutes or until the chicken is tender.

4. Add the remaining **Ingredients** and cook for additional 15 minutes. If additional water is needed in the soup, you may add ½ cup at a time.

5. Serve hot.

Nutritional Content:

Calories: 110

Potassium: 101mg

Fat: 8g

Protein: 3g

Fruity Omelette

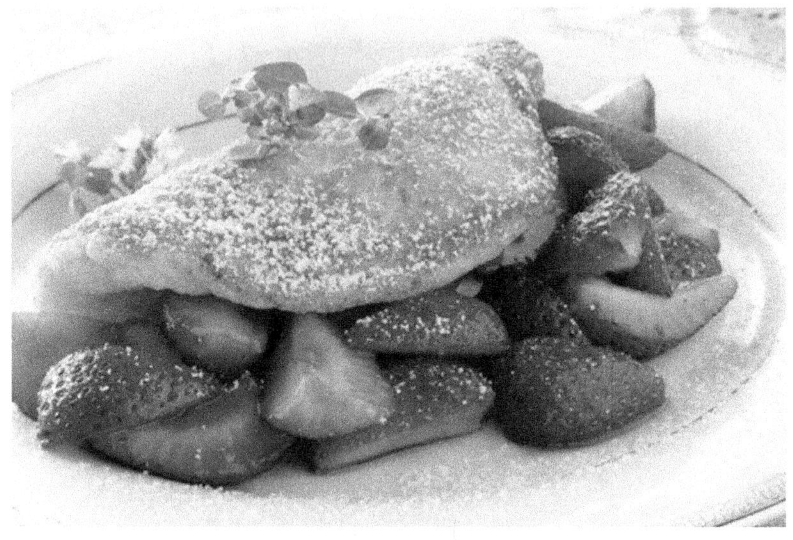

This Fruity Omelette is quick, tasty and filling.

Serves: 4

Time: 15 mins.

Ingredients

- unsweetened strawberries, 2 cups, frozen, thawed
- sugar, 1 tbsp. (optional)
- eggs, 4, separated
- lemon juice, 1 tbsp.
- butter, 1 tbsp., unsalted

Directions

1. Preheat the oven to 375ºF.

2. Now, coat your strawberries in sugar, set aside.

3. Take a medium bowl and beat the egg whites until stiff

4. Take a separate bowl and beat the egg yolks and lemon juice. Add in your stiff whipped egg whites until evenly combined.

5. Take a 10" oven-safe skillet and melt butter in it. Pour the egg mixture into the skillet. Put to cook on low heat for about 5 minutes.

6. When the mixture is place at the bottom, cook in the oven for additional 5 minutes.

7. Now, lift the omelette onto heated plate. Spoon on strawberries and cut into pie wedges.

8. Serve hot.

Nutritional Content:

Calories: 198

Potassium: 430mg

Fat: 9g

Protein: 8g

Meat Stuffed Green Peppers

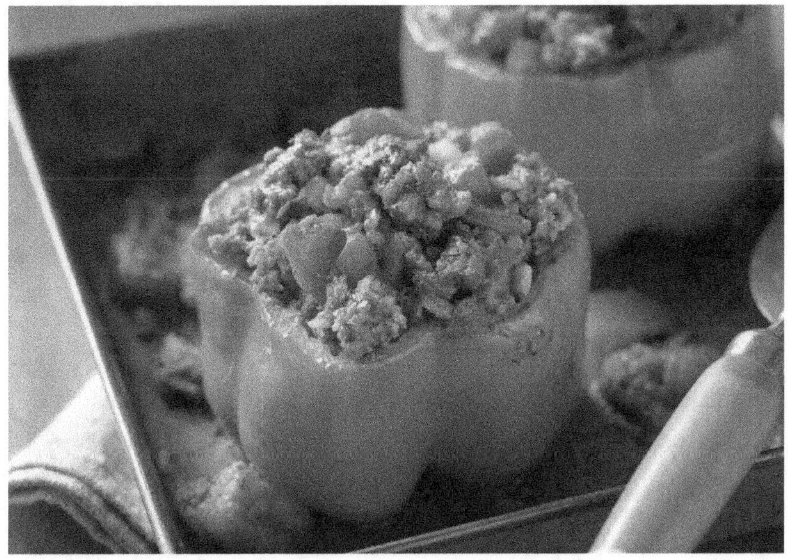

Enjoy these Stuffed Green Peppers when you need a quick, tasty meal.

Serves: 6

Time: 40 mins.

Ingredients

- vegetable oil, 2 tbsp.
- lean beef, turkey or chicken
- onions, ¼ c., chopped
- ¼ c. celery, chopped

- 2 tbsp. lemon juice

- 1 tbsp. celery seed

- 2 tbsp. Italian seasoning

- 1 tsp. black pepper

- ½ tsp. sugar

- 1 ½ c. cooked rice

- green peppers, 6, small, tops removed, seeded

- paprika

Directions

1. Preheat the oven to 325°F.

2. Heat oil then add the ground meat, celery and onions to pan, cook together until the meat is browned.

3. Now, add in your **Ingredients** except the paprika and green peppers to the saucepan. Stir together and remove from the heat.

4. Stuff the peppers with mixture.

5. Finally, wrap with the foil or place the peppers in a dish and cover. Bake the peppers for about 30 minutes. Top with paprika. Enjoy!

Nutritional Content:

Calories: 131

Potassium: 160mg

Fat: 4g

Protein: 9g

Jalapeno Pepper Chicken

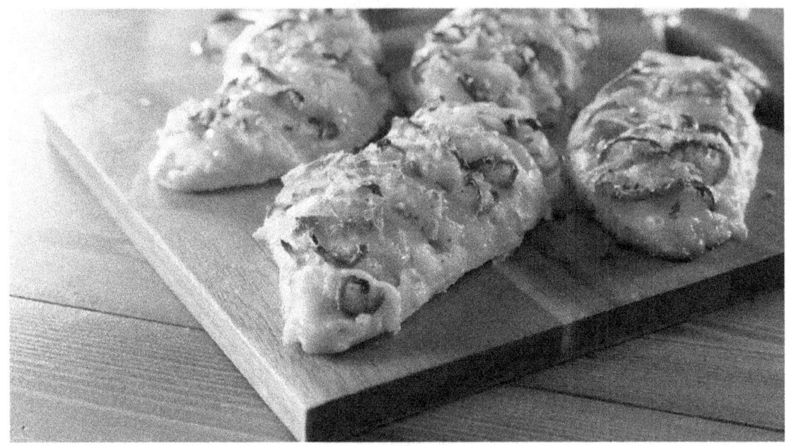

This Jalapeno Pepper Chicken has just enough spice to warm your soul with every bite.

Serves: 8

Time: 45 mins.

Ingredients

- 3 tbsp. vegetable oil
- chicken, 2-3 lbs., cut up (skin and fat removed)
- onion, 1, sliced into rings
- chicken stock, 1½ cups
- nutmeg, ½ tsp., ground
- black pepper, ¼ tsp.

- jalapeño peppers, 2 tsp., seeded, finely chopped

Directions

1. Set your oil to heat in a pan and brown the chicken pieces. Once the chicken pieces are brown, set them aside keeping warm.

2. In the same pan, sauté the onion rings. Now, add the homemade stock from cooked chicken and bring to a boil. Keep stirring in between.

3. Once the homemade stock from cooked chicken comes to a boil, add the chicken pieces, nutmeg and black pepper.

4. Cover the pan the let the chicken simmer for 30 to 35 minutes or until the chicken is tender.

5. Add jalapeño peppers to chicken and let it simmer for another minute or so. Serve hot.

Nutritional Content:

Calories: 143

Potassium: 160mg

Fat: 7g

Protein: 17g

Crispy Lemon Chicken

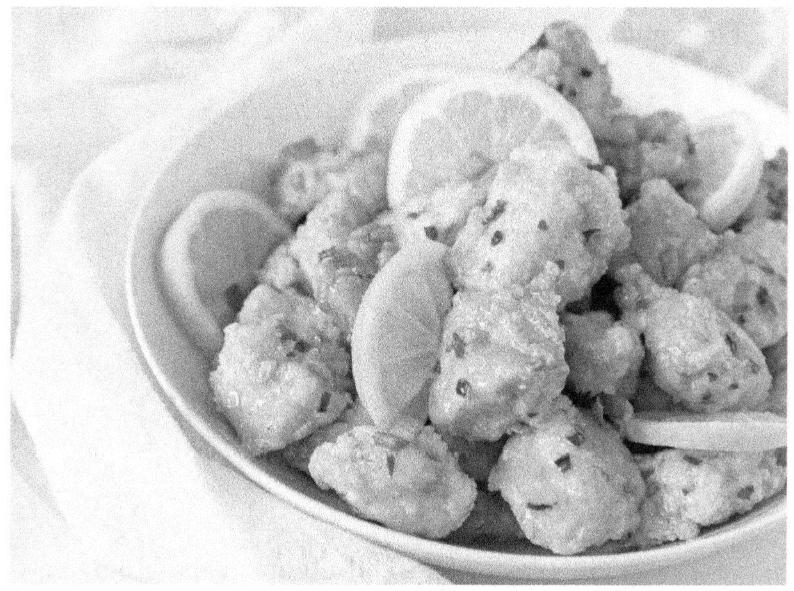

This recipe provides a tasty citrus crunch on your dinner plate.

Serves: 8

Time: 45 mins.

Ingredients

- fryer chicken, 2 ½ lb. (cut as desired)
- lemon juice, 1 tbsp.
- flour, 1 cup all-purpose

- black pepper, 1 tsp.
- corn flakes, 1 cup, crushed
- poultry seasoning, ¼ tsp.
- vegetable oil, 4 tbsp.

Directions

1. Preheat the oven to 400°F.

2. Next step is to wash, clean and pat dry the chicken pieces. Once the chicken pieces are dry, give them a bath of lemon juice.

3. Take a small plastic bag and combine the flour, corn flakes, black pepper and poultry seasoning together. Shake well.

4. Take a deep baking pan (about 1 inch deep) and grease it with vegetable oil.

5. Put the chicken in the plastic bag of **Ingredients** and shake well. Put the large pieces first followed by small ones.

6. Once the chicken pieces are well coated with the mixture, place them in the pan and brown in the oven for about 20 to 30 minutes on each side.

Nutritional Content:

Calories: 280

Potassium: 150mg

Fat: 18g

Protein: 15g

Old Style Rice and Chicken

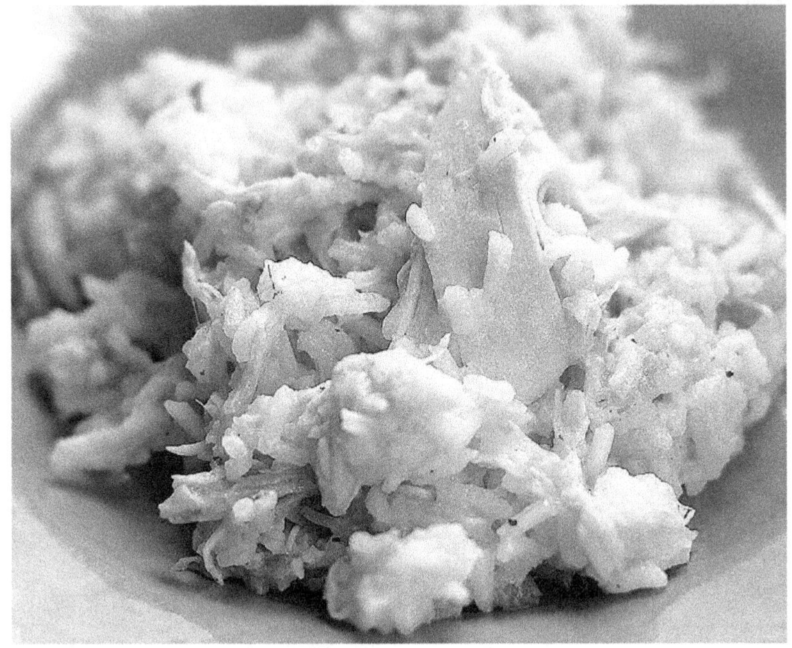

Enjoy this plate of Rice and Chicken is not only traditional but also delicious.

Serves: 6

Time: 40 mins.

Ingredients

- chicken parts, 1 lb.
- black pepper, 1 tsp.

- poultry seasoning, 1 tbsp.
- onion, ½ cup, chopped
- onion powder, 1 tsp.
- garlic powder, ½ tsp.
- bay leaves, 1 tsp., crushed (optional)
- water, 4 cups
- rice, 1 cup, uncooked
- vegetable oil, 1 tbsp.

Directions

1. Take a Dutch oven covered with water and put the chicken pieces, spring onions, onion powder, black pepper, poultry seasoning and bay leaves.

2. Cook the chicken until tender.

3. Once cooked, remove the chicken meat and skin from the bone. Keep the chicken meat but discard the skin. Also reserve 2 cups of chicken broth.

4. Take a large pot and put rice, vegetable oil, chicken meat and 2 cups of chicken broth in it. Now, bring it to a boil over medium-high heat.

5. Once it comes to a boil, reduce the heat to low and simmer for about 20 to 25 minutes.

6. Serve hot.

Nutritional Content:

Calories: 212

Potassium: 283mg

Fat: 8g

Protein: 21g

Chicken and Celery Salad

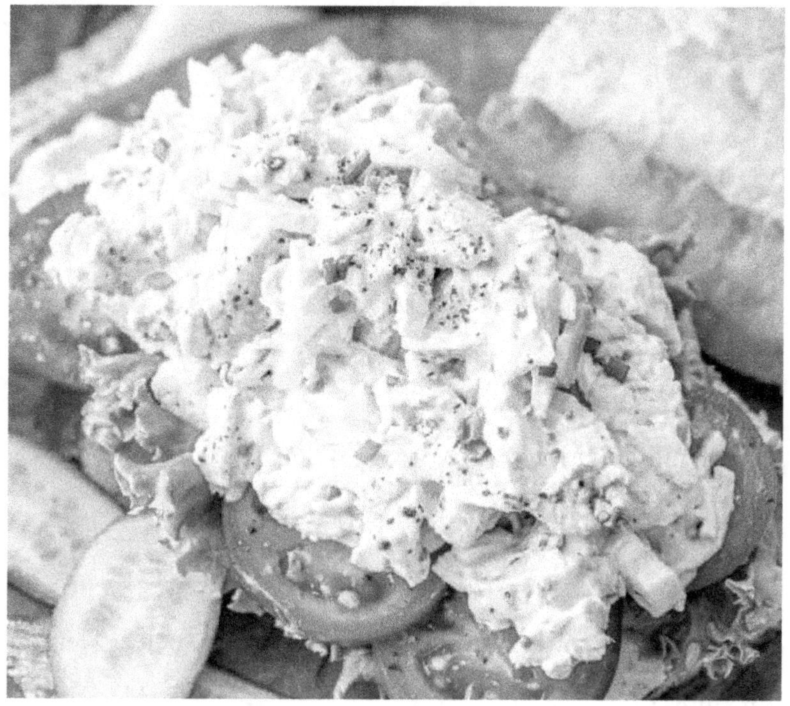

This Chicken and Celery Salad is quick to whip up and extremely tasty.

Serves: 5

Time: 10 mins.

Ingredients

- chicken, 2 c., diced
- celery, 1/3 c., chopped
- onion, ¼ c., chopped
- green pepper, ¼ c., chopped
- parsley, 1 tsp., dried (optional)
- lemon juice, 1 tbsp.
- black pepper, ¼ tsp.
- mustard, 1 tsp., dry
- mayonnaise, ½ c.

Directions

1. Take a bowl and combine chicken, parsley, celery, lemon juice and toss well.

2. Take a small bowl and combine mustard, black pepper and mayonnaise together.

3. Add the mustard mixture to chicken mixture and mix thoroughly

Nutritional Content:

Calories: 181

Potassium: 205mg

Fat: 10g

Protein: 18g

Simple Vegetables and Chicken Salad

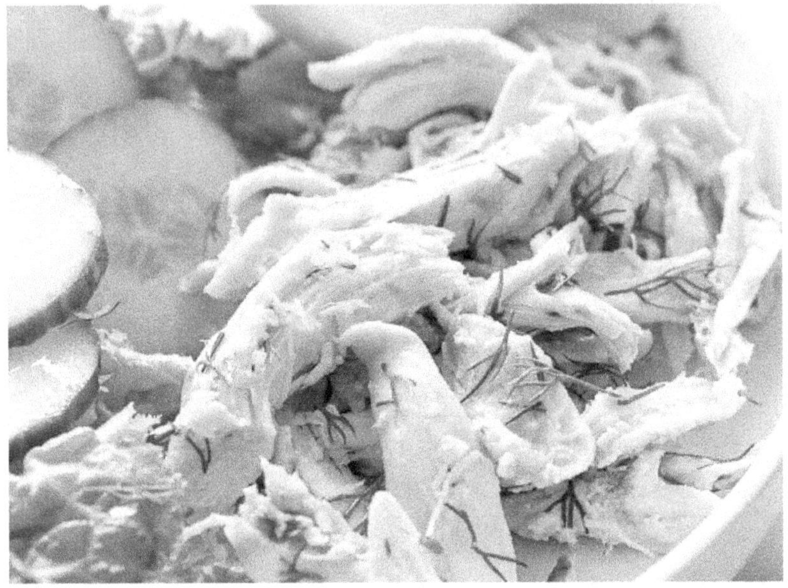

This veggie and chicken combo is super delish plus easy to whip up.

Serves: 4

Time: 10 mins.

Ingredients

- 1 ½ c. cooked chicken, diced
- ½ c. green pepper, chopped finely
- ½ c. celery, diced finely

- ½ c. onions, chopped finely
- 3 tbsp. pimentos, diced
- ½ c. salad dressing or light mayonnaise
- 1 tbsp. lemon juice

Directions

1. Take a bowl and combine chicken, spring onions, celery, and pimentos and toss well.

2. Take a small bowl and combine lemon juice and mayonnaise.

3. Add the mayonnaise mixture to chicken mixture and mix well.

4. Cover and chill in the refrigerator before serving.

Nutritional Content:

Calories: 221

Potassium: 230mg

Fat: 15g

Protein: 18g

Spring Onions and Herbs Chicken Curry

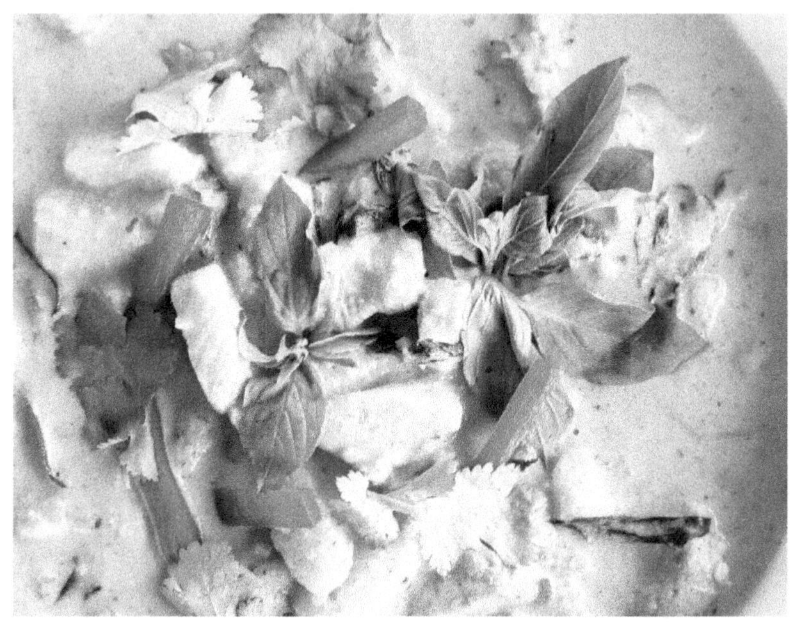

This curry is packed with flavor making delicious an understatement.

Serves: 6

Time: 2 hrs. 15 mins.

Ingredients

- chicken, 1 whole, skin removed, cut in small parts.
- lemon juice, ¼ cup

- curry powder, 2 tsp.
- onion, 1 medium, chopped
- garlic glove, 1 medium, chopped (optional)
- black pepper, ½ tsp.
- thyme, ½ tsp., dry
- olive oil, 2 tbsp.
- water, 1 cup

Directions

1. Start by cleaning the whole chicken and cut into small pieces.

2. Once you cut the chicken into small pieces, give the chicken pieces a bath of lemon juice.

3. Next, take a medium sized bowl and combine spring onions, curry powder, black pepper, thyme together. Once combined, rub the mixture onto the chicken pieces.

4. Next step is to let the chicken marinate in the refrigerator overnight or at least for 1 to 2 hours.

5. Take a saucepan and heat the vegetable oil. Sauté the marinated chicken until it turns brown.

6. Once the chicken turns brown, pour one cup of water into the pan and let the chicken simmer until it gets tender.

7. Once the chicken becomes tender, remove it from the heat and serve with hot rice.

Nutritional Content:

Calories: 323

Potassium: 317mg

Fat: 24g

Protein: 21g

Chicken and Vegetables Stew

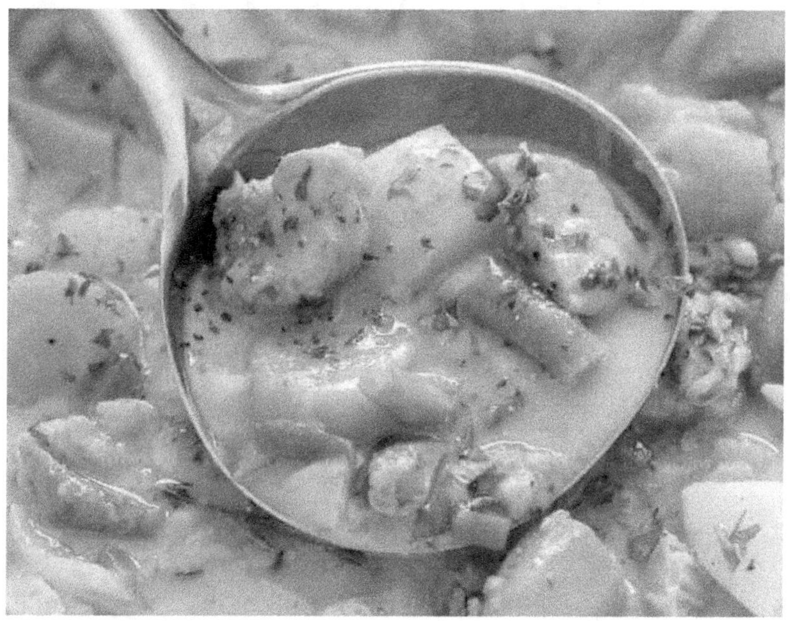

Here we have a hardy stew that is both filling and delicious.

Serves: 6

Time: 40 mins.

Ingredients

- vegetable oil, 3 tbsp.
- chicken breast, 2 lb., cut in bite size pieces
- onions, 1 c., sliced
- green peppers, ¾ c.

- garlic, 2 cloves, minced
- all-purpose flour, 2 tbsp.
- chicken broth, low-sodium, 21 oz., canned
- carrots, 10 oz., frozen
- basil, ¼ tsp., dried
- black pepper, ¼ tsp.
- okra, 110oz., frozen, sliced

Directions

1. Start by taking a Dutch oven and heating 2 tbsp. of oil in it.

2. Now, add the chicken pieces and sauté the chicken over medium-high heat.

3. Once the chicken is sautéed, remove it from the Dutch oven and set aside.

4. Now, add 1 tbsp. of oil in the Dutch oven, add and sauté the onions, garlic and pepper.

5. Now add the flour and cook it for about 2 to 3 minutes, stirring constantly.

6. Now, add the chicken and broth and cook until it boils.

7. Once the chicken broth comes to a boil, add the carrots, black pepper, and basil. Cover and let it simmer for approximately 10 to 12 minutes. The gravy will become thick as it simmers.

8. Now, add the okra and let it cook for another 5 to 10 minutes.

9. Serve with hot white rice.

Nutritional Content:

Calories: 142

Potassium: 453mg

Fat: 8g

Protein: 10g

Stir Fry Vegetables Chicken

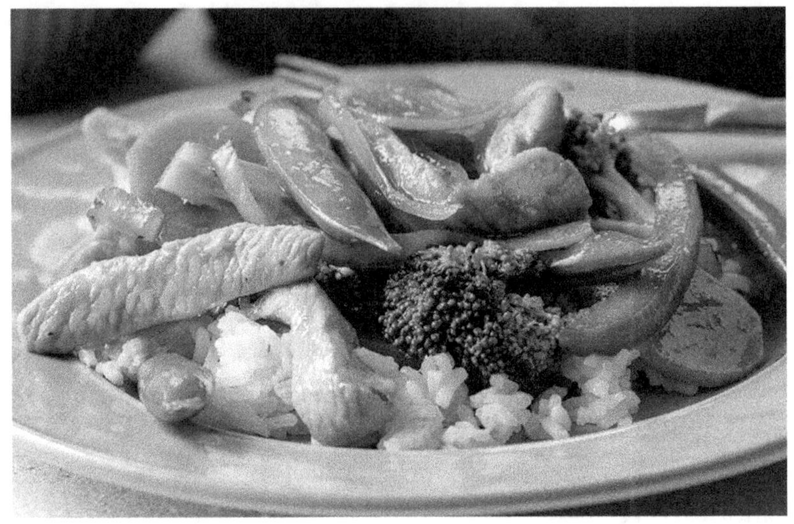

This recipe is so tasty you will be longing for more.

Serves: 3

Time: 15 mins.

Ingredients

- cooking oil, 2 tbsp.
- chicken breasts, 2, medium, diced
- stir fry vegetables, 10 oz., frozen
- liquid smoke, ½ tbsp.
- rice, 2 c., cooked

Directions

1. Take 9 to 10 inches and heat the oil on high heat.

2. Add the chicken, and sauté.

3. Stir in the vegetables.

4. Add the liquid smoke and stir everything well.

5. Reduce heat and cook uncovered for about 5 minutes, or until done, while stirring.

6. Serve over 2/3 c. of cooked rice.

Nutritional Content:

Calories: 315

Potassium: 618mg

Fat: 7g

Protein: 29g

Simple 'N' Basic Pork Chops

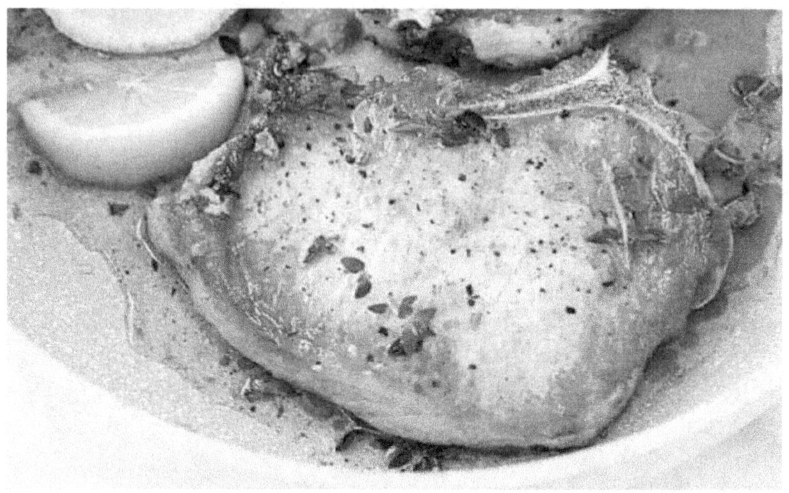

Enjoy these succulent Pork Chops over the family dinner table with all your loved ones.

Serves: 4

Time: 1 hr.

Ingredients

- vegetable oil, 2 tbsp.
- flour, ¼ cup, all-purpose
- black pepper, 1 tsp.
- sage, ½ tsp.
- thyme, ½ tsp.

- pork chops, 16 oz., lean, fat trimmed

Directions

1. Preheat the oven to 350°F.

2. Grease your baking pan well with vegetable oil.

3. Combine the flour, thyme, sage and black pepper.

4. Now dredge the pork chops in the flour mixture and arrange in the baking pan.

5. Place your pan into the oven and let the pork chops brown on both the sides. This process will take approximately 40-45 minutes.

6. Once tender, switch off heat and serve hot.

Nutritional Content:

Calories: 434

Potassium: 332mg

Fat: 34g

Protein: 19g

Pan Pork Sausage

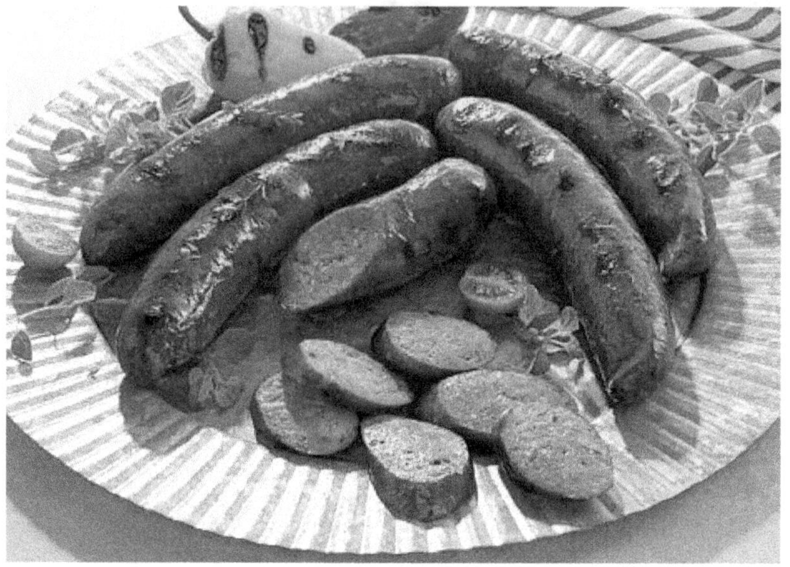

These pork sausages are perfect for lunch or dinner with your favorite sides.

Serves: 12

Time: 30 mins.

Ingredients

- ground pork, 1 lb., lean
- sage, 2 tsp., ground
- sugar, 2 tsp., granulated
- black pepper, 1 tsp., ground

- red pepper, ½ tsp., ground
- basil, 1 tsp. (optional)
- cooking spray

Directions

1. Take a large bowl and mix all the **Ingredients** well to make the sausage.

2. Once the mixture is ready, make into patties by measuring 2 tbsp. of mixture for each patty.

3. Once the patties are formed, either pan fry them or broil until they are thoroughly cooked.

Nutritional Content:

Calories: 96

Potassium: 87mg

Fat: 7g

Protein: 6g

Conclusion

Thank you for sticking with me all the way to the end of this Low Potassium Recipes Cookbook. I sincerely hope you enjoyed all 30 Healthy Low Potassium Recipes to Aid Combat with Hyperkalemia.

Feel free to leave a review on Amazon so I can know exactly what you enjoyed about our journey through our Low Potassium recipes. Then grab another one of my cookbooks for another journey.

Bye for now.